The Busy Professional's Guide to Fitness and Nutrition in 30 Minutes

Table of Contents

Chapter 1. Introduction

Introducing 'The Busy Professional's Guide to Fitness and Nutrition in 30 Minutes,' a resource that turns the perceived mountain of health into a speed bump! In this Special Report, we break down intimidating jargon into friendly, comprehensible content without skimping on the crucial elements of nutrition and fitness. You're a professional with a schedule tighter than a marathoner's new sneakers, and we know that. That's why we've tailored a guide that will help you achieve your health goals with just thirty minutes of dedication per day. No more trade-offs between meeting deadlines and living a healthy lifestyle. So gear up, because it's time to reinvent your relationship with time and wellness. Begin your delightful journey with this comprehensive guide, so you can thrive at work and beam with health every single day! Get ready for a transformation that promises to be as inspiring as your ambition!

Chapter 2. Understanding Time: Your Most Valuable Asset

Let's start by acknowledging what we've already known deep down: Your greatest ally in the quest for health and wellness isn't the newest fad diet or the latest exercise routine. It's time, that resource you're so dedicated to managing diligently at work. To thrive at work and beam with health, we need to turn towards mastering our time.

2.1. The Perception of Time

It's a funny thing, time. We set alarms to wake up, create schedules to structure our day, count down hours till the meeting, and even slip into crises mode when we fall behind. Yet it seems there's never enough of it. We're continually racing against time, often letting our health get bumped off the priority list. Why does time always seem to be in short supply?

The issue isn't that we have too little time. It's our perception of how we use, manage, and value it. Our perception of time is subjective and can be influenced by multiple factors, such as our mood, activity, culture, or even age. The perception of time can change drastically based on how engaged or interested we are in a particular activity or task. This is important to understand because it carries implications for how we can better manage our time to fit in health and wellness activities.

2.2. The Priority Matrix

Time management and prioritization often go hand in hand. It's evident that we want to dedicate time to our health, but amidst deadlines and work commitments, it somehow drops to the bottom of our to-do list. A valuable tool to aid in time management is the Priority Matrix.

The Priority Matrix categorizes tasks based on two factors: urgency and importance. Urgency signifies the time-sensitivity of a task, while importance relates to the impact it has on our objectives. The tasks are then divided into:

1. Urgent and important

2. Important but not urgent

3. Urgent but not important

4. Neither urgent nor important

By categorizing our tasks, we can attend to what's important, not just what appears urgent.

2.3. Time Blocking

Now that we understand the importance of prioritization, let's establish a practice—time blocking, a scheduling method that segments your day into blocks of time allocated for specific tasks or activities.

This segregates your day into meaningful chunks that let you focus on one thing at a time without the risk of multitasking. This method discourages distraction and promotes deep work, helping you finish tasks on time—freeing up time to engage in health and wellness activities.

2.4. Incorporating Fitness and Nutrition

With time-blocking, it becomes convenient to slot in time for exercise and balanced meals during the day—even for a busy professional. Some easy ways to incorporate it are:

1. Dedicated workout sessions: Slotting in specific periods during the day for a quick workout.

2. Meal preparations: Designating time for meal preparation goes a long way in ensuring nutritious options are available when hunger strikes during the day.

3. Short exercise breaks: These can be done during break times, and might include stretches, desk exercises, or a quick walk around the office.

4. Mindful eating: Eating slowly and without distraction, helps us consume reasonable portions and enjoy our meals more—it keeps us aligned with our nutrition goals.

2.5. Technology to the Rescue

Using technology to manage our time can make our tasks efficient and streamlined. Apps for time management, workout routines, mindfulness exercises, and nutrition tracking can help us stay on course with our health goals. Most importantly, remember to use technology to your advantage, not let it consume your time.

2.6. Time: The Intangible Asset

The 'busy' in our lives is going nowhere. But, better time management and the realization of time as the most valuable, yet intangible, asset can help us prioritize our health without compromising our professional commitments.

Integrating effective time management strategies, commitment towards prioritizing health, and helpful technological tools allow us to take control of our time. In doing so, we manage not just to survive a hectic professional life but also thrive with robust health and wellness.

Chapter 3. Demystifying Fitness: Building an Efficient Exercise Routine

When you think of the term 'fitness,' what's the first thing that pops into your mind? An elite athlete hitting the gym for hours each day? A power-lifter lifting an eye-popping weight? Or do you see a marathon runner breaking the tape at the finish line in a world-record time? While these scenarios do represent aspects of fitness, they only make up a small part of what the term truly encompasses. The foundation of fitness lies in functionality and sustainability that are interlinked with your daily life.

3.1. Your Body, The Finely-Tuned Machine

Think of your body as an automobile. Our cars require regular maintenance, the right fuel type, and sensible usage to ensure they stay in top condition. Similarly, your body needs regular exercise (maintenance), a balanced diet (fuel), and healthy habits (sensible usage) to remain in optimal health. Building an efficient exercise routine is like providing your body the regular tune-up it needs.

3.2. Understanding The Pillars of Fitness

As we delve further into the journey of designing an efficient exercise routine, let's first understand the essential components or 'pillars' of fitness: strength, cardiorespiratory endurance, flexibility, agility, and body composition.

How to incorporate all these elements into a 30-minute workout routine may seem like a puzzle. Don't worry, we will guide you through this all-important task.

3.3. Strength Training: No, You Won't Turn Into a Bodybuilder Overnight!

Contrary to popular belief, strength training isn't solely for those desiring muscle-bound physiques. In fact, it forms an integral part of any balanced fitness regimen. Strength training keeps your bones strong, boosts metabolism, and enhances functional fitness, i.e., the ability to perform daily activities comfortably.

Research suggests that even minimal resistance training can lead to significant muscular strength gains. So, how does one incorporate strength training in a 30-minute workout?

Try to allocate at least 10 minutes of your routine to this component. Include exercises like push-ups, squats, lunges, and planks. Start with one set each, gradually increasing as your strength improves. Don't forget about your safety: form over number of reps should be your guiding principle here.

3.4. Cardio: You Don't Have to Run a Marathon to Boost Your Heart Health

Cardio, short for cardiovascular activity, alludes principally to exercises that increase heart rate. These could range from activities like brisk walking, cycling, jumping jacks or even climbing stairs. The goal is to enhance your body's oxygen utilization, thus improving heart health and endurance.

In a 30-minute exercise routine, aim for 10-15 minute spread of cardio activities. You could break them into smaller chunks or use High-Intensity Interval Training (HIIT) to get the maximum benefits. Remember, the key to cardio is consistency, not intensity; therefore, choose a form that you enjoy and can sustain daily.

3.5. Flexibility and Agility: Stretch and Move Your Way to Better Health

Why are flexibility and agility significant? Well, they enable us to move easily, maintain balance, and avoid injuries. These are especially crucial as we age, with our body gradually losing its suppleness.

To incorporate flexibility and agility into your 30-minute routine, opt for exercises like light yoga or dynamic stretching for about 5 minutes. This can be done either at the beginning (as a warm-up) or the end (as a cool down) of the workout.

3.6. Body Composition: Why It Matters?

Body composition refers to the proportion of fat, muscle, bones, and water in the body. Maintaining a healthy body composition reduces the risk of diseases like obesity, diabetes, and heart diseases. While specific body composition goals differ from person to person, it is generally healthier to have more muscle than fat.

You can influence your body composition with a sound dietary plan coupled with strength training and consistent cardio activities. Remember, an efficient 30-minute exercise routine is just one part of the equation; a balanced, nutrition-rich diet is the other.

3.7. Crafting Your Routine

Now that we have understood the pillars of fitness, let's look into constructing an efficient 30-minute routine. Consider alternating strength and cardio days, with flexibility exercises included every day. Begin every session with a warm-up and end with a cool-down. Listen to your body, adjusting the intensity depending on how you feel on a particular day.

An example routine might look like this:

- Day 1: Strength training (10 minutes), Cardio (15 minutes), Flexibility (5 minutes)
- Day 2: Cardio (15 minutes), Strength Training (10 minutes), Flexibility (5 minutes)
- Day 3: Rest or Light Activity
- Day 4: Repeat

Remember, the goal is to build a routine that is efficient, sustainable, and enjoyable. Start with small, realistic steps, gradually increasing intensity and complexity as your fitness level improves.

Maintaining the efficiency of your routine can happen only when combined with proper nutrition, rest, and stress management. Remember, this journey of fitness is not a sprint, but a lifelong marathon. So take your time, enjoy the process, and let the transformation happen naturally!

Finally, don't forget to consult a healthcare or fitness professional if you have any underlying medical condition that you are concerned about. They can guide you through building the right fitness routine, taking into account your medical needs, fitness level, and personal goals. Every individual's journey to fitness is unique; make yours something to remember!

Chapter 4. Nutrition 101: Fuel Your Body Right Without the Fuss

Nourishing your body is like fueling a vehicle. You wouldn't stuff candy into your car's gas tank, so why inundate your body with less-than-quality nutrition?

4.1. Understand the Importance of Balanced Diet

A balanced diet is your body's fuel station, where you fetch sustenance for the long journey of life. It isn't just about weight management; it also significantly affects your mood, energy, and even cognitive functions. Consuming a balanced mix of carbohydrates, fats, proteins, vitamins, and minerals ensures your body is well-equipped to function optimally.

Packing your meals with plenty of fruits, vegetables, lean proteins, whole grains, and low-fat dairy products, while curtailing your intake of sodium, saturated and trans fats, and added sugars, can have some powerful health perks. Lower risk of chronic diseases, improved bodyweight control, and better physical and mental health are just a few benefits of eating right!

4.2. The Building Blocks of Nutrition: Macronutrients and Micronutrients

Macronutrients are the body's bulk fuel suppliers. They comprise carbohydrates (our primary energy source), proteins (crucial for tissue repair and growth), and fats (our energy storage solution). On the other hand, micronutrients are vitamins and minerals that perform hundreds of roles in the body despite being needed in minuscule amounts.

- **Carbohydrates** provide 4 calories per gram, but not all are created equally. Opt for complex types found in whole grains over simple ones found in sugary foods.

- **Proteins**, also delivering 4 calories per gram, are best derived from lean sources like fish, poultry, beans, lentils, and low-fat dairy.

- **Fats** pack a punch at 9 calories per gram. Prioritize unsaturated fats found in oily fish and olive oil and minimize saturated fats found in full-fat dairy and takeaway meals.

As for micronutrients, an all-inclusive multivitamin can bridge any small gaps in your diet.

4.3. Building Your Healthy Plate

Building a healthy, balanced plate is simpler than you might think. Here's a simple rule-of-thumb guide to get you started:

- Fill half your plate with colorful fruits and vegetables. These fiber, vitamin, and mineral powerhouses not only fuel your body but also make your meals visually appealing.

- Designate a quarter of your plate for whole grains like brown rice, barley, or whole grain bread. These complex carbs deliver slow-release energy, keeping you satisfied longer.

- Fill the remaining quarter of your plate with lean protein sources. This can be white meat, fish, or plant-based options like legumes and tofu.

- Don't forget to include a source of healthy fats on your plate;

think avocado, nuts, seeds, or a drizzle of extra virgin olive oil.

4.4. Meal Planning and Prepping: A Busy Professional's Best Friend

Learning to meal prep effectively can save not just your precious time but also your health. Here's how:

1. Pick a day of the week when you have a few hours to spare for meal prep.

2. Plan your menu for the week ahead, considering variety and balance.

3. Make a grocery list according to your meal plan to avoid impulse purchases.

4. Cook and portion out your meals in reusable containers.

By spending a few hours one day a week prepping your meals, you can ensure you have nutritious food ready at all times.

4.5. Smart Snacking: Fueling Between Meals

Snacks, chosen wisely, can help maintain energy levels between meals and even contribute to your daily nutrient intake. So, incorporate healthy snacks, such as fruits, yogurt, nuts, and seeds, helping keep those energy levels up while staying on track with your nutrition goals.

4.6. Hydration: The Often-Forgotten Nutrient

Adequate hydration is also key to optimal health. Aim for about 8 glasses of water per day, but remember, needs can vary based on age, sex, pregnancy, and exercise levels.

Taking control of your diet doesn't have to be an uphill climb. When you're informed and proactive, you can enjoy delicious meals that fuel your body properly and still meet your professional deadlines.

So, adopt these nutrition practices today for the benefit of your health – think of it as the fuel that will power your journey to the top!

Chapter 5. Morning Masterclass: Kick-Start Your Day the Healthy Way

Before the hustle and bustle of your day begins, the very first activity in the morning can set the tone for the rest of your day. We understand how precious your time is, and so, we have curated an all-encompassing plan that perfectly balances fitness and nutrition, designed to maximize your well-being in just 30 minutes each morning.

5.1. Seize the Day with Healthy Hydration

The first thing you should do after awakening is to hydrate yourself, as dehydration can sap your energy and impede concentration. During your sleep, you essentially go without water for about 7-9 hours, so drinking water first thing in the morning is key to kick-start your metabolism.

To practice this efficiently, keep a bottle of water by your bedside every night, so you can drink it as soon as you wake up. In 2-3 minutes, you've fired up your metabolic engines and are good to move onto the next step.

5.2. Wake Up and Stretch

A brief session of stretching can increase your circulation after a night of rest. The advantage of morning stretching is it's a gentle and friendly way of reminding your muscles they have a full day of activity ahead.

Invest 5-7 minutes in stretching exercises, focusing on your major muscle groups like shoulders, neck, back, and legs. Practices like yoga with its variety of asanas can be beneficial and invigorating for the body.

You don't need to solely rely on traditional stretches. Pilates exercises, such as "the hundred", which is a core-focused movement, can enhance your stamina and help you energize your whole body.

5.3. Eye of the Tiger - Quick High Impact Workout

The key here is a high impact yet condensed workout. You want to get your heart rate up and get in that sweet spot where you're sweating and breathing hard, but not absolutely out of breath. This ensures that you're pushing yourself to your body's peak performance in a limited timeframe.

Choose routines like High-Intensity Interval Training (HIIT) or circuit training that can maximize the effectiveness of your workout in a minimum amount of time. A basic HIIT routine can look like this:

1. Warm up - Light jogging in place (1 minute)

2. High knees - Running in place, bringing your knees up to your chest (1 minute)

3. Jumping jacks (1 minute)

4. Burpees (1 minute)

5. Rest (30 seconds)

Repeat this circuit three to five times, dependent on your comfort level. Keep this for a span of 14-16 minutes, and you will feel energized for the day.

5.4. Power-Shower and Preparing for the Day

A quick shower after your workout can be very refreshing. Not only does it cleanse your body, but it also helps to wake you up fully and revitalize your senses. This step can take you around 5-7 minutes.

Whilst showering, you can mentally prepare for the day ahead, perhaps mentally going through the tasks you have at hand or simply focusing on the feel of the water, practicing a little mindfulness.

5.5. Breakfast, The King of Meals

The term "breakfast" means to break the fast that occurred while you were sleeping, and it's considered as the most important meal of the day. A well-balanced, nutritious breakfast fuels your body for the day and aids in maintaining a healthy weight.

Our recommendation for a power-packed breakfast in 10-12 minutes includes a serving of whole grains, a source of lean protein, fruits or vegetables.

An example might be an egg-white omelet with spinach, cherry tomatoes, and a slice of whole-grain bread on the side. Or, for a vegan alternative, try a generous bowl of oatmeal topped with berries and a splash of almond milk.

By the time you're done, you've spent around 30 minutes actively managing your health.

Making these aspects of your morning routine ensures you've put your best foot forward for the day ahead. This Morning Masterclass is designed to slot seamlessly into your busy schedule, not as an extra task, but a part of your lifestyle so that you can thrive in your personal and professional life. Incorporate these methods into your routine and watch as your days become more productive, energetic, and focused.

Chapter 6. Effective Breaks: Fitness Tactics for Busy Days

Embracing fitness in the midst of busy days often poses a challenge. Nevertheless, integrating wellness activities into the daily hustle bustle is not only doable but also essential. Effective breaks that prioritize fitness can transform these seemingly mounting challenges into opportunities for stress relief, refreshment, and renewed focus. Let's dive deep into how to make the most of these breaks during hectic days.

6.1. Making the Most of Short Breaks

Short breaks may not seem like much, but they can be a goldmine for increases in productivity and fitness levels. Just a few minutes can be designated to engage in exercises that amplify strength and flexibility.

Defining a short break would typically refer to a span ranging from 5 to 15 minutes. In this mini window, you can engage in multiple exercises, including desk-based ones.

For instance, you may want to begin with some neck rolls, attempting to rotate your neck before moving onto wrist and ankle rotations. The 'seated leg raiser', 'book press', and 'desk chair swivel' are other exercises conceivable from the comfort of your office chair.

Cap off your short breaks with a simple walk; this can be as uncomplicated as visiting the washroom or walking to the water dispenser. Remember, this is about making the most of every spare minute you have during your busy day.

6.2. The Power of Mid-Length Breaks

Mid-length breaks are usually around the 15 to 30 minutes mark. Here, your options extend far beyond desk-based exercises, although they can still be beneficial.

Try a brisk walk around your workplace or if you work from home, spend this time walking outside for some fresh air. Walking helps to improve cardiovascular health, increases stamina, and can even improve your mood. Other options can include stair climbing, which is a great aerobic exercise that strengthens the leg muscles.

Make use of app-based workouts. There are numerous fitness apps available designed specifically for short, intense workout sessions. You may want to explore apps that direct exercises, such as the 7-minute workout. This enables you to venture into a collection of exercises that challenge numerous muscle groups within that designated timeframe.

6.3. Unleashing the Potential of Longer Breaks

Finally, we move onto longer breaks, typically ranging from 30 minutes to 1 hour. These spans present you with an optimal chance to indulge in a series of workouts that stretch beyond the comforts of your workplace or home office.

During this interval, you can take a yoga or Pilates class, or at least part of one. Both of these options are fantastic for flexibility and core strength without overly elevating heart rate – great if you've got to get right back to work afterward.

Working out in a gym is also viable if you have one nearby. A series of machines and free weights enable varied exercises, which is beneficial for both cardiovascular and strength training.

The final consideration can be running. Running promotes heart health and burns considerable calories, making it a worthwhile consideration if your schedule and location accommodates it.

6.4. The Art of Deskercises

Deskercise is a compound of two words: desk and exercise, and refers to exercises that you can do right at your desk. This is fantastic news for professionals who find themselves glued to their desks the majority of the day. A few minutes of stretching, followed by exercises aimed at strengthening muscles, can work wonders.

Examples include seated leg raises, chair squats, desk push-ups, and seated torso twists. Regularly engaging in these exercises not only increases your fitness level but also reduces the risk of health issues such as obesity, high blood pressure, and diabetes.

6.5. Balancing Nutrition on Busy Days

No fitness guide would be complete without acknowledging the crucial role that nutrition plays on busy days. Prioritizing your dietary needs during breaks is as important as incorporating physical activity.

Remember to hydrate, eat frequent small meals, and avoid excessive consumption of caffeine and sugars. Opt for protein-rich foods with ample fruits and vegetables. Balancing your diet goes a long way in augmenting the fitness efforts you integrate into your daily routine.

6.6. Making It a Lifestyle

Ultimately, fitness on busy days boils down to lifestyle changes. It involves integrating wellness activities into the daily flow, and creating habits that are sustainable in the long run. This might mean waking up earlier to get in a workout, taking the stairs instead of the elevator, choosing salad over fast food, or squeezing in a couple sets of deskercises in between meetings.

Remember, every step counts, even if it seems small at first. As you form healthier habits, these small steps will cumulate and lead to noticeable changes in your fitness and overall well-being, ensuring that you can thrive both professionally and personally.

Chapter 7. Meeting with Meals: Eating Healthy on the Go

We live in a world where convenience often markets unhealthy food as your best friend. But don't worry, with the right tactics and a shift in mindset, you can turn the tables around and conquer your nutrition goals, even when you're pressed for time. This chapter will guide you on how to navigate the tricky waters of eating healthily on the go, while keeping it simple and straightforward.

7.1. The Art of Meal Preparation

Meal preparation, a term that you've probably encountered if you've dipped your toes into the fitness world, is your secret weapon for retaining control over your diet when time is sparse.

It refers to the practice of preparing and cooking meals ahead of time, usually for the upcoming week. This strategy is effective as it saves you time on busy days, eliminates the risk of making unhealthy dining choices when pressed for time, and can help save money too.

Take some time during the weekend, or any free timeslot you can carve out, to plan, purchase, and prepare your meals for the coming days.

- Decide on a menu that includes meals covering breakfast, lunch, dinner, and two smaller snack batches meant for mid-morning and mid-afternoon.

- Ensure these meals are balanced with a good mix of proteins, carbohydrates, and fats. Including a variety of fruits and vegetables would deliver your much-needed fiber and micronutrient quotas.

- Invest in good-quality airtight containers for storing meals.

The goal is to make meals that are not just healthy, but also flavorful, to keep your taste buds interested. Remember, it's not just about eating to live, but savouring the process too.

7.2. The Smart Grocery Shopping Guide

Even the best-laid meal prep plans can go astray if you end up with an empty pantry. Effective grocery shopping is an art that requires a little bit of strategic planning.

Stick to these principles when you're shopping for groceries:

- Make a list and stick to it. A list ensures you don't forget key ingredients and helps ward off impulse purchases.

- Shop primarily in the outer aisles of the grocery store. This is usually where the fresh produce, lean meats, dairy, and whole grain products are stocked.

- Read labels. Make sure you're getting products that are low in added sugars, high in fiber, and free from processed ingredients.

- Don't shop hungry. This can lead to impulse purchases of unhealthy foods.

7.3. Snacking Intellectually

For a busy professional, smart snacking can serve as a bridge between meals, helping to maintain stable blood sugar levels and stave off extreme hunger that often results in overeating.

Here are a few smart snacking tips for busy professionals:

- Plan your snacks just like you plan your meals.

- Keep a range of healthy snacks at your workplace and pack some in your bag for the day.

- Great options include nuts and seeds, fresh or dried fruits, yogurt, hummus, and baby carrots.

- Skip the sugary drinks. Opt for water, herbal teas, or green teas for hydration.

7.4. Dine-out Options: Making Healthy Choices

If you're a professional, chances are that eating out is inevitable at times. But that doesn't mean your health goals have to take a hit. Here's how you can continue eating healthy even when dining out:

- Opt for grilled, baked, or broiled meats instead of fried.

- Choose restaurants that offer healthier choices and provide calorie counts on the menu.

- Be cautious of calorie-laden dressings, sauces, and dips.

- Opt for water or unsweetened beverages, rather than sugary drinks and alcoholic concoctions.

- Practice portion control. If the portions are large, consider packing half to take away.

Your relationship with food amidst your busy schedule doesn't have to be a tricky compromise anymore. With practical strategies that involve meal preparation, smart grocery shopping, intellectual snacking, and making healthier choices when dining out, this chapter equips you to embrace a nutritious diet even when on the run. Purposefully take one step at a time and soon enough, you'll master the art of eating healthy on-the-go. After all, the true spirit of a professional is in not giving up, and that applies to your health journey too.

Chapter 8. Stay Hydrated: The Unassuming Key to Energy and Focus

We need to discuss the simplest yet most overlooked component of our personal health and wellbeing — water. This vital nutrient plays an essential role in maintaining energy levels, enhancing focus, and promoting overall body functioning. Despite its significance, it's all too easy for busy professionals to lose sight of proper hydration.

8.1. Understanding Hydration

Our bodies are about 60 percent water; our brains, close to 80 percent. Every cell, tissue, and organ in our body relies on water for survival. It's no wonder that even slight dehydration can significantly disrupt physiological functions and lead to fatigue, impaired cognition, and decreased concentration.

To ensure optimum health and vitality, it's vital to maintain an ideal water balance in the body. Each day our body loses fluid through breathing, sweating, and digestion, and it's essential to replenish these water losses. The National Academies of Sciences, Engineering, and Medicine has suggested a daily fluid intake of approximately 3.7 liters (or about 13 cups) for men and 2.7 liters (or about 9 cups) for women. These amounts include all beverages and food, but keep in mind that the optimal amount varies depending on your weight, activity level, and climate.

8.2. The Impact of Dehydration on Energy Levels

Ever wondered why you feel lethargic during the day, especially in the afternoon? You might attribute it to having a big meal, too little sleep, or stress. However, mild dehydration is a common culprit. Even a fluid loss of 1-2% can impair cognitive performance, leading to feelings of fatigue, mood changes, and a decrease in alertness and concentration.

In fact, the body's physical performance can also be drastically affected. It impedes cardiovascular function and limits the body's ability to dissipate heat, thus decreasing endurance and increasing fatigue. This becomes particularly important if your work involves any physical activity or if you maintain a regular exercise routine.

8.3. Hydration for Enhanced Focus

Proper hydration is not just about preventing fatigue. It plays a crucial role in maintaining focus and attention, too. When the body is well-hydrated, there is an adequate blood volume that circulates oxygen and essential nutrients to the brain, stimulating cognitive functioning.

Studies show that even mild dehydration can impair a range of cognitive functions, including attention, motor coordination and complex problem-solving skills. So next time when you're preparing for that crucial presentation, remember to have a water bottle at hand!

8.4. How to Stay Hydrated

For busy professionals, it can be a real challenge to keep up with hydration needs. One effective way to ensure you're drinking enough water throughout the day is to incorporate it into your routine:

- Start your day with water: Tie it to a daily ritual, like brushing your teeth. Because you'll have gone many hours without any fluid intake during sleep, your body will appreciate the immediate hydration.

- Have a drink with every snack and meal: Incorporating a beverage can also aid in digestion.

- Keep a water bottle at your workplace: A visual reminder goes a long way in ensuring you stay hydrated.

- Utilize technology: Various phone apps not only remind you to drink water but also keep track of how much you've consumed and how much more you need to fulfill your daily quota.

Remember, not all fluids have the same hydrating power. While beverages like coffee and tea do contribute to your overall water intake, they also have a diuretic effect, which can lead to increased fluid losses. Sweetened drinks add unnecessary calories and often fail to quench your thirst as effectively as water.

8.5. Looking Beyond Water

Hydration isn't just about guzzling water. In fact, around 20% of our daily fluid requirement comes from solid foods. Many fruits and vegetables like melon, cucumbers, and strawberries are high in water content. Incorporating these into your daily meals can supplement liquid intake and offer a range of other essential nutrients.

Sports drinks can be helpful for those engaging in long-duration high-intensity workouts. They replenish electrolytes lost in sweat, but for most people's activity levels, drinking sufficient amounts of water and maintaining a balanced diet should suffice.

In conclusion, as a busy professional, the simple act of maintaining proper hydration can do wonders for your performance and productivity. Prioritize this overlooked element in your daily routine. After all, water is the fuel that runs the engine of your body, and staying hydrated is the key to keeping the engine optimal.

Chapter 9. A Good Night's Sleep: The Underrated Powerhouse

Sleep, though often overlooked, is an essential key to optimizing your health and maximizing your performance both at work and physically. A peaceful, restful slumber can amplify your cognitive abilities, improve your mood, and give your body the much-needed energy to take on whatever the day brings. By understanding the science of sleep and incorporating a few techniques into your routine, you can master the art of a good night's sleep.

9.1. Understanding the Science of Sleep

The human body operates on a 24-hour cycle known as circadian rhythm. This internal clock controls many physiological processes, including body temperature, hormone release, and – you guessed it – sleep. Sleep itself can be divided into two kinds: Rapid Eye Movement (REM) sleep and Non-REM sleep. Non-REM sleep consists of three stages, the final stage being deep sleep. It's during this deep sleep and the REM sleep cycles where rejuvenation occur.

Each night, a typical sleep pattern will cycle between Non-REM and REM sleep several times. Both are crucial, with Non-REM sleep playing a part in memory consolidation and REM sleep stimulating the regions of the brain used in learning. In other words, a productive day begins with a good night's sleep.

9.2. The Impact of Sleep on Health and Fitness

Consistent, quality sleep leads to a stronger immune system, better heart health, increased productivity, improved mood, and even weight loss. Sleep deprivation, on the other hand, can have serious consequences for your health and performance.

- **Immune Function**: Your immune system uses sleep as a time to rest and rebuild. Shorting yourself on sleep can leave you susceptible to infections and prolong your recovery time when you do get sick.

- **Mental Performance**: A sleep-deprived mind lacks the ability to concentrate, make decisions, and react quickly. This can significantly hamper your work performance.

- **Emotional Well-being**: Chronic lack of sleep can lead to mood swings and increase the risk of depression and anxiety.

- **Physical Health**: Sleep deprivation has been linked to chronic diseases like diabetes, heart disease, and obesity.

9.3. Regulating Your Internal Clock

Synchronizing with your body's natural circadian rhythms can improve sleep quality and overall health. Regular sleep schedules, exposure to natural light, and maintaining a sleep-friendly environment are simple ways you can fine-tune your internal clock.

1. **Consistency is key**: Establishing a consistent sleep schedule can help reinforce your body's sleep-wake cycle. Try to keep the same sleep schedule on weeknights and weekends.

2. **Manage light exposure**: Daylight is a powerful stimulator of the circadian rhythm. Try to get outside in natural light for at least a half-hour each day.

3. **Create a restful environment**: Keep your sleep environment dark, quiet, cool, and free from distractions. Consider using eye shades, earplugs, or a white noise machine if needed.

9.4. Optimizing Pre-Sleep Habits

Equally as important as the sleep itself are the habits around sleep – your sleep hygiene. Small changes to your pre-sleep routine can have significant impacts on your sleep quality.

- **Dinner choices**: Heavy, rich meals close to bedtime can cause discomfort and disrupt sleep. Also, limit caffeine and alcohol, both well-known sleep disruptors.

- **Unplug**: The blue light emitted by screens can interfere with your sleep cycle. Make screen-free time a part of your pre-sleep routine.

- **De-Stress**: Relaxation exercises, such as progressive muscle relaxation, deep breathing, mindfulness, can help signal to your body that it is time for sleep.

9.5. The Power of Napping

While the focus of this chapter is on a good night's sleep, it's worth noting that short naps during the day can also contribute to your rest and recovery. A 20-30 minutes nap can provide a much-needed boost of alertness and cognitive functioning.

9.6. The Next Steps: Monitoring and Adjusting

Keep a sleep diary to monitor your sleep patterns and identify potential disruptions. Self-monitoring along with these insights about sleep science and hygiene practices, can go a long way towards optimizing your sleep and, in turn, your health and productivity.

Remember, everyone is unique, and responses to various techniques may differ. Experiment with different strategies to learn what works best for you, and most importantly, respect your need for a good night's sleep. It's not time wasted, but time invested in health, wellness, and productivity.

Chapter 10. Maintaining Balance: Holistic Approach to Mental and Physical Health

Establishing balance is crucial in not just achieving physical health but also securing mental wellbeing. Your body and mind operate together as a unit; when one is out of sync, the other often follows suit. In this chapter, we will explore the holistic approach to maintaining your mental and physical health for overall wellbeing, unravelling tips and advice along the way.

10.1. The Foundation: Understanding Holistic Health

Holistic health sees the body, mind, and spirit as a unified entity that needs to be in balance. This perspective regards any imbalance (physical, emotional, or spiritual) as disruption to your overall health.

A holistic approach involves various elements such as proper diet, physical activity, sleep and rest, along with mental exercises like meditation and mindfulness. You don't need to excel in one and neglect the others - it's about finding a balance that makes you feel good and function optimally.

10.2. The Physical Aspect: Nutrition and Exercise

Nutrition relates directly to your physical health. A well-balanced diet fuels your body for everyday tasks, providing the energy and nutrients necessary for cell growth and repair. Consuming a variety of foods from different food groups is key:

- Protein: Builds and repairs tissues
- Carbohydrates: Primary energy source
- Fats: Supports cell growth
- Vitamins and minerals: Essential for various bodily functions
- Fiber: Aids digestion

Regular exercise diminishes the risk of developing chronic diseases, improves mood, helps control weight, enhances sleep, and increases energy levels. It doesn't have to be overly intensive; even brisk walks or daily stretches can significantly impact your health positively.

10.3. The Mental Aspect: Stress Management and Mindfulness

Undue stress has detrimental effects on both your mental and physical health, manifesting in various forms such as headaches, sleep disorders, weight gain, and, in severe cases, heart disease. Hence, effective stress management techniques are paramount. A popular one is mindfulness - the practice of staying fully in the present moment without judgment.

Mindfulness teaches you to recognize stressful thoughts and emotions, understand their transitory nature, and let them pass without getting overwhelmed. Regular practice promotes mental resilience, reducing stress, anxiety, and depression.

10.4. The Spiritual Aspect: Meditation and Connection

Spiritual health refers to having a purpose in life and feeling connected to a greater whole. Meditation is a popular practice that encourages spiritual health, helping to calm the mind and deepen the connection with oneself. Regular practice can lead to reduced stress, improved focus, and enhanced empathy.

Moreover, fostering a connection with others through community activities or volunteering can also improve mental wellbeing, leading to feelings of satisfaction and fulfillment. Finding time for such activities within a busy schedule may be challenging, but remember, even small interactions can have profound effects on your wellbeing.

10.5. Putting it All Together: Strategies for a Balanced Approach

The first step is to acknowledge that mental and physical health are intertwined, and both need attention. Incorporate small changes gradually into your life instead of trying to overhaul your entire lifestyle at once.

Create a weekly plan that includes a balanced diet, regular exercise, mindfulness, and social interaction. Keep the plan flexible to suit your work schedule and personal preferences. Setbacks are inevitable, but remember: progress, not perfection, is the goal.

Remember, the journey towards holistic health is personal and unique. The balance that works for one may not work for another. By understanding and applying the principles of holistic health, you can navigate your way towards a healthier, happier life. It's not merely about adding years to your life but adding life to your years.

The holistic approach, wrapped in its broad context, is precisely the encompassing perspective that busy professionals need. By catering to the various dimensions of your health, you not only ensure physical vitality but also warrant a sound and peaceful mind. With a commitment of just thirty minutes a day, this balanced worldview can be both attainable and sustainable.

Chapter 11. Sustaining the Habit: Keeping your Momentum in the Long Run

Your journey towards better fitness and nutrition doesn't end once you've established a routine; in fact, maintaining your momentum is an integral part of this journey. This can often feel as though you're crossing an endurance-testing mountain range, but with the right tools and mindset, you can transform this challenge into a manageable daily practice.

11.1. Mastering Your Mindset

In order to sustain your fitness routine and nutritional habits, you first need to grapple with your mindset. Your thoughts profoundly influence your abilities to maintain a course of action. Therefore, it's essential to foster a positive mindset, one which encourages persistence and resilience.

A key component of a powerful mindset is the firm belief in your ability to succeed. This belief, often termed as "self-efficacy," forms the foundation upon which the habit building stands. Foster this conviction, continually affirm that no matter the obstacles, you have the ability and determination to maneuver your way through to reach your fitness and nutrition goals.

To strengthen self-efficacy, set attainable goals. While it's understandable to aim for the moon, it's also important to find a balance between setting challenging and attainable goals. Starting with smaller, achievable goals boosts your self-confidence and motivates you to tackle more significant challenges.

11.2. Creating a Support System

Even with unwavering determination, there will be days when your energy will be low, and motivation on the decline. These periods are normal and an anticipated part of the journey. A well-constructed support system can be greatly beneficial during such times.

A support system can comprise people who share similar goals, friends, family, or health professionals. These individuals can be your cheerleaders, providing encouragement when you need it the most. They could also benefit from learning about your aspirations, getting inspired in the process to adopt healthier routines themselves.

Moreover, consider hiring a certified coach or subscribing to digital fitness platforms to get professional guidance. They can provide personalized advice and novel methods to keep you engaged and on track.

11.3. Tracking Progress and Celebrating Success

A simple yet effective method to maintain momentum is to keep track of your progress. Documenting your journey serves a dual purpose – It lets you see how far you've come and who you're becoming.

Consider utilizing fitness apps that can track your exercise routines, calories intake, sleep patterns, and more. These statistics are excellent motivators that can also help you tweak your plans as required.

Last but not least, celebrate your success. Rewarding yourself when you attain a milestone, no matter how small, reinforces the positivity associated with the efforts you've put in. These rewards shouldn't contradict your fitness and nutrition goals; instead, they should be things that elevate your well-being and boost your motivation.

11.4. Nutrition for Sustenance

An indispensable aspect of maintaining your momentum is offering your body the proper nutrition it needs. The right foods can fuel your body, enhance performance, accelerate recovery, and even uplift your mood.

Understand that there's no 'one-size-fits-all' when it comes to nutrition. Hence, it is beneficial to consult with a nutrition professional to find a diet plan that suits your lifestyle, food preferences, and fitness goals. They can assist you in making informed decisions about portion control, balanced nutrition, and timing of meals.

Keep in mind, a nutritious diet does not mean depriving your taste buds. In fact, it's quite the opposite. There's a plethora of nutritious and delicious food choices available, and knowing what to eat empowers you to make healthier choices that also satisfy your palate.

11.5. Dealing with Setbacks

In your journey towards a healthier lifestyle, there will be days or even periods of setbacks. It's crucial to understand that this is completely normal. Remember, progress is measured in resilience and perseverance rather than perfection. It's about embracing the ups and downs and learning how to rise after the fall.

When faced with a setback, don't beat yourself up. Instead, regroup and re-strategize. Try and identify what led to the setback and devise a plan to tackle it in the future.

11.6. Listening to Your Body

Your body is constantly communicating with you, sending signals about what feels good and what doesn't. Developing the habit of listening to these signals often assists you in maintaining the momentum in the long run.

Endeavor to discern signals of true hunger, fatigue, and stress. Do not ignore the signs of discomfort during any physical activity, as they may lead to serious injuries. It's completely alright to ease up and rest when needed. Remember, recovery is as essential as the workout itself.

By keeping these aspects in mind, you are well on your way to build and maintain momentum. It's a journey about continuous learning, adapting, and taking care of yourself. It is about celebrating every little win and never forgetting why you started. By doing so, you will find that the journey towards an integrated fitness and nutrition lifestyle becomes enriching, rejuvenating, and worthwhile.